Chair Yoga for Seniors Over 60

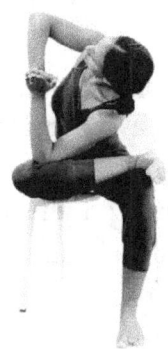

The Easy Step-by-Step Guide with Low Impact Exercises to Reclaim Balance, Mobility and Lose Weight in 10 Minutes Per Day

Stacey R. Smith

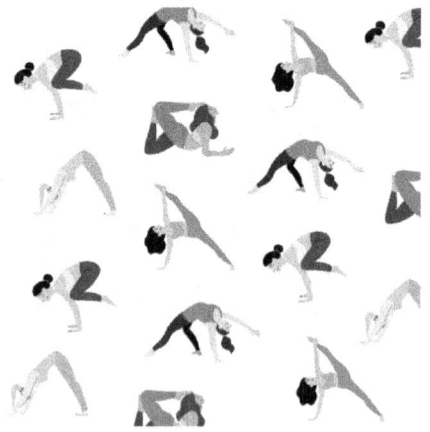

TABLE OF CONTENTS

Free Gift For You!

Don't miss out on the transforming power of our **"Wall Pilates Workouts for Women"**. Click to embark on a fitness adventure that combines the benefits of Pilates with simple wall workouts. Achieve results in only minutes each day and up your fitness game!

What will I benefit by going through this book?

• An approach to holistic fitness
• Focused Wall Exercises
• Time-effective and Easy-to-Achieve Exercises
• Transformative Results

INTRODUCTION

Agnes McTavish, my next-door neighbor, used to be as nimble as a cricket. Even though her oven hadn't seen flour in years, she filled the air with the familiar smells of cinnamon and bread. Age, on the other hand, had taken its toll. Agnes limped along the corridor, her back bent like a question mark, her once sparkling eyes dulled with concern. She'd fallen twice in the previous month, and the prospect of another slip was eroding her confidence.

The delicious aroma of baking was replaced one morning by the steady thud of a cane. I peered out and saw Agnes doing tai chi in her doorway, imitating a hummingbird video on her tablet. "Morning, Agnes!" I said. "Trying a new routine?"

Her giggle was a scratchy rasp that made my heart skip a beat. "I'm doing my best, darling. Gravity seems to have it in for me these days."

That's when the thought occurred to me. I dashed back to my apartment and retrieved my long-forgotten book of "Chair Yoga for Seniors Over 60." I returned to Agnes, tucking it under my arm. "Mind if I give you something?"

Agnes' brow furrowed as she received the book, her attention fixed on the title. "What about chair yoga? Sounds impressive for resting on my backside."

I smiled. "Certainly not! Gentle stretches and motions may be done straight from your chair. Perfect for people like us."

That day marked the start of a wonderful friendship. We began with easy exercises, with Agnes seated in her favorite recliner and me on the floor leading her through the positions. We'd take in the early light, arching our arms like sunflowers towards the sky, chuckling at our shaky efforts. Agnes gradually changed in front of my eyes. Her slumped back straightened, her feet grew lighter, and she regained a cheeky twinkle in her eyes.

"You know, dear, this book isn't just about the exercises," Agnes said one afternoon. "It is all about hope. It reminds me that even at my age, I can exercise and feel powerful."

Her words warmed me like a hot croissant. My book, which I had written out of a desire to help people, had found its ultimate purpose in Agnes' living room. It wasn't only about restoring balance or losing weight; it was also about rediscovering the joy of movement, the spark of independence, and the unshakeable spirit that age couldn't fade.

Agnes became my yoga cheerleader as the weeks evolved into months. We'd have morning meetings in the corridor, our motions attracting the attention of other inhabitants. A motley bunch of elders soon joined us, changing the corridor into a makeshift yoga studio full of laughing, moans, and the steady creak of chairs.

Agnes, once imprisoned by fear, became the heart of our small community. Her voice was hoarse but warm, and her eyes twinkled with humor as she led basic breathing exercises. She even persuaded Mr. Henderson to join us, his scoffs replaced by hesitant smiles as he found the unexpected strength in his aged legs.

Agnes stroked my hand as we sipped tea after our lesson one crisp autumn morning. "Thank you, dear," she murmured, her voice full of love. "You gave me more than just my equilibrium back. You restored my pleasure."

I gazed about at the circle of happy faces, the early sun painting golden squares on the floor. My book had grown from a collection of words on paper to a bright tapestry of optimism, connection, and the quiet defiance of age. And it all began with a simple act of compassion, demonstrating the transformational potential of a little chair yoga and a lot of human love.

Agnes' narrative and our chair yoga practices became a beacon of light in our small world. It reminded us that even the tiniest act of kindness may create a wave of happiness that impacts lives in unexpected ways. Agnes, on the other hand, is the uncontested queen of our chair yoga team, her contagious joy and newfound confidence showing that even at the age of ninety, life is still full of possibilities waiting to be embraced, one gentle stretch at a time.

Why Choose Chair Yoga?

Chair yoga is a modified form of conventional yoga in which the practitioner sits on or uses a chair for support. It is useful for people who have mobility concerns, low flexibility, or find it difficult to practice yoga on the floor. Chair yoga incorporates moderate stretches, breathing exercises, and relaxation methods, making it suitable for elderly, office workers, and those healing from ailments. It can aid in the improvement of flexibility, balance, and general well-being.

Common Chair Yoga Fallacies

1. Only for Seniors or People with Limited Mobility: One of the most common misunderstandings is that chair yoga is just for elders or those with restricted mobility. While chair yoga has many benefits for these populations, it is also appropriate for people of all ages and physical abilities. It may be tailored to different fitness levels and even used as a supplement to regular yoga practice by emphasizing alignment, breath, and awareness.

2. Chair Yoga Isn't a Real Workout: Some people wrongly feel that chair yoga isn't a real workout because it requires sitting. Chair yoga, in actuality, may be rather strenuous. It works several muscle groups, increases flexibility, and enhances balance. Many chair yoga sequences include postures, stretches, and motions that challenge the body and enhance cardiovascular health. It may not be as intense as high-impact workouts, but it provides a distinct and beneficial kind of physical activity.

3. Ineffective for Stress release and Relaxation: The effectiveness of chair yoga to offer stress release and relaxation is frequently underestimated. People may believe that only conventional yoga on a mat may give these advantages. Chair yoga, on the other hand, involves mindfulness, deep breathing, and relaxation methods, which can help decrease tension and anxiety. It is an easy approach to practice mindfulness and find moments of tranquility while sitting.

4. Chair Yoga Has a Limited Variety of Postures and Movements: Some people say that chair yoga is restrictive and only offers a limited variety of postures and movements. Chair yoga, on the other hand, is extremely adjustable and adaptive. It may be altered to incorporate a broad range of postures, stretches, and motions that target various muscle groups and enhance flexibility. To add diversity and difficulty to chair yoga sessions, instructors frequently utilize props such as tension bands or tiny weights.

5. Not Beneficial for Overall Well-Being: Chair yoga is frequently viewed as a kind of exercise without taking into account its comprehensive advantages. Aside from physical fitness, chair yoga has other benefits for general well-being. It has the potential to improve posture, circulation, mood, and contribute to improved sleep. The emphasis on breath awareness and mindfulness in the practice might improve mental clarity and emotional equilibrium.

6. Limited Audience: Another myth is that chair yoga is only good for a small group of people. In reality, chair yoga can benefit a wide range of people, including office workers looking to relieve desk-related tension, people recovering from injuries, pregnant women seeking gentle movement, and anyone looking to incorporate movement into their daily routine without requiring a mat or open space.

7. Lack of Challenge and Intensity: Some people wrongly believe that chair yoga is less challenging and intense than conventional yoga. While chair yoga may be tuned to deliver a surprisingly difficult exercise, it can also be reduced for softness. Skilled instructors create sequences that include dynamic movements, resistance exercises, and bodyweight exercises, ensuring that participants use their muscles and raise their heart rates.

8. Inadequate for Improving Flexibility: A widespread misconception is that chair yoga does not help with flexibility. Chair yoga, contrary to popular thought, contains a range of stretches and positions that progressively build flexibility. Participants focus on increasing their range of motion while keeping their body's limits in mind, which helps to prevent accidents and enhance joint health.

9. Not a "Real" Yoga Practice: Some purists believe that chair yoga isn't a "real" yoga practice since it deviates from traditional mat-based practice. Chair yoga, on the other hand, honors the notion that yoga is ultimately about the unification of body and mind. It adjusts yoga poses and concepts to diverse physical demands, making it a genuine style of yoga just like any other.

10. Minimal Mind-Body Connection: Another common misperception about chair yoga is that it lacks the mind-body connection associated with conventional yoga. In actuality, chair yoga emphasizes breath awareness, mindfulness, and meditation. Participants are instructed to link their breath to movement, fostering inner quiet, self-awareness, and mental clarity.

11. Unsuitable for Weight reduction Goals: Although chair yoga does not burn as many calories as high-intensity workouts, it can still help with weight reduction and control. Regular chair yoga practice can boost metabolism, promote mindful eating, and foster a healthy relationship with one's body. Furthermore, the stress-relieving benefits of chair yoga might indirectly help weight reduction by lowering emotional eating.

The beliefs that underpin chair yoga's adaptability, efficacy, and inclusion are the source of its flaws. By refuting these beliefs, we identify chair yoga as a useful practice that provides individuals of varied abilities and requirements with physical health, mental clarity, emotional balance, and a deeper feeling of well-being. As with any kind of exercise, approaching chair yoga with an open mind and a desire to investigate its possible advantages is critical.

CHAPTER 1: UNDERSTANDING THE BENEFITS OF CHAIR YOGA

Understanding the benefits of chair yoga is critical for seniors looking for a gentle yet effective way to improve their overall well-being. Chair yoga, a modified form of conventional yoga, has several physical, mental, and emotional benefits that are specifically adapted to the requirements of those over the age of 60.

Chair yoga improves flexibility, allowing seniors to regain and maintain their range of motion. Chair yoga postures relieve stiffness with moderate motions and stretches, especially in areas prone to pain or arthritis. Flexibility improves not just daily activities but also minimizes the chance of injury by improving balance and coordination.

Chair yoga is a strong technique for stress reduction and relaxation, both mentally and emotionally. The practice of mindful breathing methods and meditation helps to maintain a calm and focused mind. Seniors frequently have lower levels of anxiety and a greater capacity to regulate stress, which contributes to better mental health.

Chair yoga is also suitable for elders with various levels of mobility. Individuals feel empowered when they participate in activities tailored to their ability. This openness is critical for cultivating a good mentality and motivating elders to continue their fitness quest.

Chair yoga provides a sense of community and social connection in addition to physical and emotional advantages. Group chair yoga classes allow seniors to engage, share experiences, and encourage one another on their wellness path. This social element is critical in battling feelings of isolation and loneliness, which are frequent issues for older persons.

To summarize, comprehending the advantages of chair yoga entails realizing its comprehensive influence on the physical, mental, and emotional health of seniors. Seniors may recapture their energy, encourage relaxation, and develop a supportive community by adopting this adaptive and accessible type of exercise, all of which contribute to a more meaningful and active lifestyle in their golden years.

Physical Benefits

Chair yoga is a type of yoga that can be done while seated on a chair, making it an accessible and useful exercise for seniors. Below are some of the physical benefits of chair yoga for seniors:

1. Improved Flexibility And Range Of Motion:
Chair yoga postures gently stretch and mobilize the muscles and joints, which can assist to improve flexibility and range of motion. This can make it simpler to do everyday tasks like getting dressed, reaching for things, and climbing stairs.

2. Increased Strength And Balance: Chair yoga postures also assist to strengthen the muscles, which can enhance balance and coordination. This can assist to lower the risk of falls, which are a big worry for seniors.

3. Reduced Pain And Stiffness: Chair yoga can help reduce pain and stiffness in joints such as the knees, hips, and back. This is because the positions increase circulation and flexibility.

4. Improved Cardiovascular Health: Chair yoga can enhance cardiovascular health by boosting heart rate and circulation. This can assist to increase overall fitness and minimize the risk of heart disease.

5. Improved Mental Health: Chair yoga can also improve mental health. The gentle movements and emphasis on the breath can help to relieve tension, anxiety, and sadness.

6. Improved Sleep: Chair yoga can also aid with sleep quality. The relaxation methods employed in chair yoga might assist in preparing the body for sleep.

In addition to these physical benefits, chair yoga may be an enjoyable and sociable exercise for seniors. There are several chair yoga sessions offered in community centers, senior centers, and yoga studios. These programs can give a chance for seniors to meet new people, mingle, and have fun while remaining active.

Mental and Emotional Benefits

Aside from the physical benefits of increased flexibility, strength, and balance, chair yoga has a wealth of mental and emotional benefits for seniors. Let's take a closer look at how this gentle activity might improve your well-being:

1. Stress and Anxiety Reduction:

• **Mindful Movements and Focused Breathing:** Chair yoga stresses slow, controlled motions that are synchronized with deep breaths. This attentive practice activates the parasympathetic nervous system, causing the production of calming substances like GABA and serotonin, which help to alleviate stress and anxiety.

• **Distraction from Problems:** Focusing on the present moment via yoga poses draws your attention away from daily troubles and ruminations. This brief vacation might bring much-needed mental relief.

2. Better Mood and a More Positive Outlook:

• **Endorphin Boost:** Chair yoga, like any other physical activity, causes the release of endorphins, the body's natural feel-good chemicals. These endorphins improve your mood, making you feel more hopeful and pleasant.

• **Sense of Accomplishment:** Mastering new positions and having your body move more easily can be quite empowering. This sense of success enhances self-esteem and promotes a more optimistic attitude on life.

3. Improved Concentration and Cognitive Function:

• **Mind-body Connection:** Chair yoga emphasizes matching breath with movement, which promotes a greater mind-body connection. This increased awareness can help with attention and concentration, which benefits cognitive performance.

• **Reduced Cognitive Decline:** According to research, regular yoga practice can help prevent the start and progression of age-related cognitive decline, such as Alzheimer's disease and dementia.

4. Encourages Relaxation and Better Sleep:

• **Deep Breathing Techniques:** The emphasis in chair yoga on deep, diaphragmatic breathing promotes the relaxation response, decreasing the heart rate and soothing the nervous system. This improves sleep quality by easing you into a relaxed state.

• **Reduced Pain and Discomfort:** The gentle stretches and postures of chair yoga can help reduce joint pain and stiffness, resulting in a more pleasant night's sleep.

5. Increases Social Connection and Reduces Loneliness:

• **Group Sessions:** Attending chair yoga classes allows for social interaction with peers, which can help elders overcome feelings of loneliness and isolation.

• **Sense of Belonging and Community:** The shared experience of practicing yoga together may promote a sense of belonging and community, which can improve emotional well-being.

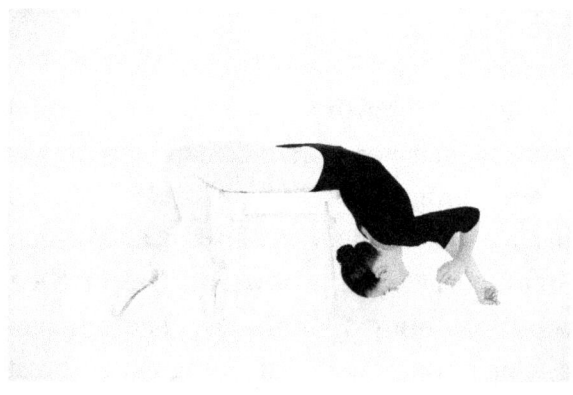

CHAPTER 3: BREATHING TECHNIQUES FOR RELAXATION AND STRESS REDUCTION

Chair yoga is a gradual road to better physical health for many elders. However, its advantages extend well beyond the physical, into the realms of mental health and emotional equilibrium. Breathwork is one of the most powerful techniques in our transforming toolbox.

Breathing methods, which are simple yet effective, may be smoothly incorporated into chair yoga sessions, opening the door to relaxation and stress reduction. So, elders, take a deep breath and be ready to exhale your anxieties!

Why is Breathing Important?

Before we get into particular strategies, let's first grasp why breath is so powerful. The mind-body link is built on our breath. When we are anxious, our breathing becomes shallow and fast, which causes our nervous system to go into overdrive. Slow, regulated breaths, on the other hand, stimulate the parasympathetic nervous system, causing the production of soothing chemicals and ushering in a state of relaxation.

Chair yoga breathing has a relaxing impact that extends beyond the exercise. Incorporate these tactics into your regular life anytime you sense stress beginning to seep in. While standing in line, feeling overwhelmed at home, or simply enjoying a calm time, take a few slow, deep breaths. Allow your breath to serve as an anchor, an inner shelter in the midst of life's storms.

So, elders, embrace breathwork's transformational potential. You set the road for a calmer, more peaceful, and joyous existence with each focused inhale and exhale. Breathe comfortably, breathe deeply, and breathe your way to a happy, healthier you.

Importance of Breath in Chair Yoga

It is impossible to overestimate the significance of breath in chair yoga for elders, since the practice's foundation is mindful breathing, which has many health and psychological advantages catered specifically to the requirements of the elderly.

Mindful breathing is a means of entering a state of calm. Seniors frequently deal with pressures brought on by changes in society, health issues, or life transitions. Deep, deliberate breathing techniques are emphasized heavily in chair yoga, which triggers the body's relaxation response. This reduces stress in the short term and enhances mental health in the long run by encouraging serenity and calmness.

Breathing with awareness improves circulation by increasing oxygenation throughout the body. Seniors who practice chair yoga breathing methods improve oxygen delivery to critical organs and tissues. This increase in oxygen delivery promotes vitality and helps maintain cardiovascular health in general. It can also lead to an increase in energy, which helps fight weariness.

In chair yoga, breath awareness is also essential for controlling pain and discomfort. Many elderly people suffer from age-related illnesses or chronic disorders. Chair yoga assists people in being more conscious of their bodies and how they respond to discomfort by combining targeted breathing techniques. Seniors who experience this increased awareness may learn how to regulate and lessen their discomfort, which will give them a sense of empowerment and control over their physical health.

Moreover, there is a strong correlation between mindful breathing and enhanced cognitive performance. Blood that is high in oxygen promotes brain health by improving mental functions including attention, concentration, and memory. For seniors who want to keep their mental sharpness and stave off cognitive loss, this is especially important.

Breath awareness also functions as a focus point for mindfulness and meditation in the context of chair yoga. Seniors are urged to focus on their breathing and to be fully present in the moment. In addition to fostering inner serenity, this meditation practice lowers stress and increases emotional fortitude.

The significance of breath in chair yoga for older citizens goes beyond simple breathing. It is an effective technique for mindfulness, oxygenation, pain relief, relaxation, and improved cognitive function. Seniors may enjoy a comprehensive approach to well-being, fostering both physical and mental vigor in their daily lives, by implementing mindful breathing into their practice.

Step-by-Step Breathing Exercises

1. Diaphragmatic Breathing (Abdominal Breathing):

• Find a comfortable chair and sit with your feet flat on the floor.
• Place your hands on your abdomen and chest.
• Inhale gently through your nose, allowing your abdomen to rise.
• Feel your air extend to your lower lungs, pushing your hands outward.
• Exhale softly through your lips, feeling your abdomen constrict.

• Concentrate on the rise and fall of your abdomen while moving your chest as little as possible.
• Repeat for 5-10 breaths, gradually increasing the time.

2. Equal Breathing (Sama Vritti):
• Sit comfortably with your back straight.
• Inhale four times through your nose.
• Hold your breath for four counts.
• Exhale through your nose for another four counts.
• Maintain a steady pace while gradually raising the count to six or eight.
• Aim for a balanced length of inhalation, retention, and exhale.

3. Box Breathing (Square Breathing):
• Sit or relax comfortably.
• Inhale four times through your nose.
• Hold your breath for four seconds.
• Exhale gently through your lips for a count of four.
• Hold your breath for another four counts.
• Repeat the cycle, increasingly prolonging each step.

4. Alternate Nostril Breathing (Nadi Shodhana):
• Sit comfortably, with your spine stretched.
• Close your right nostril with your thumb.
• Inhale from your left nostril.
• Close your left nostril with your right ring finger, releasing the right nostril.
• Exhale via the right nostril.

• Inhale via the right nostril, shut it, and exhale through the left.

• Continue in this alternate pattern for numerous cycles.

5. Resonant Breathing:

• Sit or lay down comfortably.

• Inhale deeply through your nose while counting to four slowly.

• Exhale loudly with pursed lips for the same count.

• During exhalation, concentrate on producing a calm "ocean wave" sound.

• Repeat for 5-10 minutes, changing the tempo as needed.

6. Guided Visualization Breathing:

• Find a peaceful place and close your eyes.

• Inhale deeply through your nose, envisioning a bright, good energy entering.

• Exhale through your lips, imagining tension and negativity departing.

• Incorporate calming hues or serene scenes into your vision.

• Repeat for 5-10 breath cycles, allowing the mind to completely engage.

7. 4-7-8 Breathing (Relaxing Breath):

• Sit or lay down comfortably.

• Inhale softly for four counts via your nose.

• Hold your breath for a count of seven.

• Exhale thoroughly through your mouth for a count of eight.

• Repeat for 4 cycles, progressively increasing with practice.

8. Lion's Breath (Simhasana Pranayama):
• Sit cross-legged or in a chair.
• Inhale deeply through your nose.
• Exhale forcefully through your mouth, extending out your tongue and generating a "ha" sound.
• Repeat for 5-10 breaths, relieving tension and encouraging face relaxation.

9. Kapalabhati (Skull-Shining Breath):
• Sit comfortably with your back straight.
• Take a deep inhalation through your nose.
• Exhale firmly while squeezing your abdominal muscles.
• Inhale gently, allowing the breath to enter spontaneously.
• Begin with 10 fast breaths and eventually build to 20 or more.

10. Progressive Relaxation Breathing:
• Sit or lie down in a comfortable position.
• Inhale deeply and gently, tensing your toes as you do so.
• Hold the strain for a few seconds, then exhale softly, releasing the tension in your toes.
• Continue this cycle, working your way up through each muscle group.
• Finish by tensing and releasing face muscles for a full relaxation cycle.

Incorporating Mindful Breathing into Daily Life

Incorporating mindful breathing into daily life is a transformational practice that extends the advantages of conscious breathing beyond dedicated sessions, incorporating serenity and presence into many elements of one's routine. Here's a step-by-step method to incorporating mindful breathing into your daily routine:

1. Morning Rituals:

• As you wake up, start your day with focused breathing.

• Before getting out of bed, spend a few seconds inhaling deeply and gently exhaling.

• Connect with your breath to establish a pleasant tone for the day ahead.

2. Commute Mindfully:

• Use your commute, whether driving or taking public transit, to practice mindful breathing.

• During red lights or breaks in your route, pay attention to your breathing.

• Tune in to your breath sensations to ground yourself in the middle of the daily hustle.

3. Work Breaks:

• Incorporate small focused breathing breaks during your workplace.

• Close your eyes for a few minutes, inhale deeply, and exhale gently.

- Reset your concentration and reduce stress to boost overall productivity.

4. Mealtime Awareness:

- Practice mindful breathing before meals to promote appreciation and awareness.
- Take time to breathe and exhale, taking in the nutrients before you.
- Eat gently, mindfully relishing each bite.

5. Mindful Walking:

- Incorporate attentive breathing throughout your everyday walks.
- Coordination your breath with your steps, generating a pattern of intake and exhale.
- Bring your attention to the feelings of walking and breathing in unison.

6. Technology Breaks:

- Use screen breaks to practice mindful breathing.
- Step away from your electronics, close your eyes, and take several deep breaths.
- Release stress and refocus before returning to your work.

7. Routine Before Sleeping:

- Before going to bed, try some conscious breathing.
- Lie down comfortably, focus on your breathing, and let go of the tension of the day.
- Make a peaceful transition to a comfortable night's sleep.

8. Waiting Mindfully:
• Accept waiting times as opportunities for awareness.
• Use the time you're in line or waiting for an appointment to reconnect with your breath.
• Convert idle periods into peaceful interludes.

9. Mindful Interactions:
• Engage in attentive breathing throughout talks.
• Take a deep breath before answering to encourage active listening and meaningful conversation.
• Develop a sense of presence in your encounters.

10. Nature Connection:
• Spend time in nature and combine mindful breathing with the great outdoors.
• Deeply inhale the fresh air, taking in the beauty of your surroundings.
• Allow nature to serve as a backdrop for your focused breath awareness.

Individuals may create a continuous sense of calm, attention, and awareness by integrating mindful breathing throughout these diverse aspects of everyday life. The practice continues beyond official sessions, becoming a vital part of one's lifestyle, boosting general well-being and resilience in the face of life's obstacles.

CHAPTER 4: JOINT PAIN EXERCISES

1. Seated Neck Stretch

• Sit comfortably with your feet flat on the floor.
• Inhale and stretch your spine.
• Exhale while gradually bending your head to one side and moving your ear toward your shoulder.
• Hold for 15-30 seconds, feeling a stretch down the side of your neck.
• Repeat on the opposite side.

2. Wrist Circles

• Extend your arms in front of you, palms down.
• Rotate your wrists in a clockwise and counter-clockwise manner.
• Make 10 circles in each direction.
• This exercise improves wrist mobility and relieves joint pain.

3. Ankle Rolls

• Lift one foot off the floor and spin your ankle in a circular manner.
• Perform 10 circles in one direction, then switch.
• Rep with the opposite foot.

• Ankle rolls increase ankle flexibility and decrease stiffness.

4. Seated Cat-Cow Stretch

• Sit with your spine straight and your hands on your knees.
• Inhale while arching your back and elevating your chest (Cow pose).
• Exhale while rounding your spine and bringing your chin to your chest (Cat pose).
• Repeat this flow for 1-2 minutes to lubricate the spine and relieve lower back pain.

5. Chair Forward Bend

• Sit on the edge of the chair, feet hip-width apart.
• Inhale and stretch your spine.
• Exhale, hinge at the hips, and extend forward toward the floor or your shins.
• Hold for 15-30 seconds, experiencing a nice stretch down your spine and hamstrings.

6. Seated Knee Lifts

• Sit tall with your feet level on the floor.
• Lift one knee toward your chest, holding it with both hands.

• Hold for a few breaths, experiencing a mild stretch in your hip.
• Lower the foot and repeat on the other side.
• This exercise increases hip and knee flexibility.

7. Seated Twist

• Sit with your feet flat on the floor.
• Inhale, stretch your spine, and shift your body to one side.
• For a deeper stretch, place your opposite hand on the outside of the knee.
• Hold for 15-30 seconds before switching to the other side.
• Twisting improves spinal mobility and alleviates lower back discomfort.

8. Seated Leg Extension

• Sit with your back straight and one leg out in front of you.
• Flex your foot and hold for 15-30 seconds.
• Repeat with the other leg.
• This exercise stretches the hamstrings and improves joint flexibility.

9. Seated Hip Opener

• Sit with your back straight and your right ankle crossed over your left knee.
• Gently press down on your right knee, experiencing a stretch in the outer hip.
• Hold for 15-30 seconds before switching to the other side.
• This position relieves stress in the hips and lower back.

10. Seated Shoulder Rolls

• Sit comfortably with your feet flat on the floor.
• Inhale and elevate your shoulders towards your ears.
• Exhale and roll your shoulders back and down.
• Repeat this motion for 10-15 times.
• Shoulder rolls serve to relieve stress and increase mobility in the shoulder joints.
Perform these chair yoga exercises on a daily basis, paying attention to your breath and avoiding any movements that create pain. Before beginning a new workout plan, consult with a healthcare practitioner, especially if you have pre-existing joint problems.

CHAPTER 5: ENHANCING MOBILITY

1. Seated Side Stretch

• Sit tall with your feet level on the floor.
• Inhale and extend your arms upwards.
• Exhale and slowly tilt to one side while keeping your hips planted.
• Hold for 15-30 seconds, feeling a stretch down your side.
• Inhale back to the center and repeat on the opposite side.

2. Chair Leg Swings

• Sit on the edge of the chair, feet hip-width apart.
• Hold onto the chair for support.
• Swing one leg forth and backward, gradually increasing the range of motion.
• Perform 10 swings on each leg.
• This workout increases hip mobility and flexibility.

3. Seated Torso Twist

• Sit with your feet flat on the floor and your back straight.

• Inhale and stretch your spine.
• Exhale and twist your torso to one side, holding onto the back of the chair.
• Hold for 15-30 seconds, experiencing a stretch in your spine.
• Inhale back to the center and repeat on the opposite side.

4. Seated Knee-to-Chest Stretch

• Sit with your feet flat on the floor.
• Lift one knee toward your chest, holding it with both hands.
• Hold for 15-30 seconds, experiencing a stretch in your hip.
• Lower the foot and repeat on the other side.
• This exercise improves hip flexibility and range of motion.

5. Chair Squats

• Stand behind the chair, feet hip-width apart.
• Hold on to the back of the chair for support.
• Inhale and bend your knees, lowering your hips towards the chair.
• Exhale and push through your heels to return to a standing position.
• Repeat for a total of 10-15 squats.

• Chair squats increase hip mobility and leg strength.

6. Seated Hip Circles

• Sit tall with your hands on your knees.
• Inhale, elevate your right knee, and circle it clockwise.
• Exhale, drop the knee, and circle counterclockwise.
• Repeat for 5 rounds in each direction, then transfer to the left leg.
• This workout improves hip joint mobility.

7. Ankle Alphabet

• Raise one foot off the floor.
• Use your big toe to "write" the alphabet in the air.
• Perform the alphabet in both clockwise and counterclockwise ways.
• Switch to the opposite foot.
• Ankle alphabets increase ankle mobility and flexibility.

8. Seated Forward Fold

• Sit with your feet flat on the floor.
• Inhale and stretch your spine.

• Exhale, bend at the hips, and extend forward with your hands.
• Hold for 15-30 seconds, experiencing a stretch down your spine and hamstrings.
• Return to an upright position by inhaling.

9. Seated Shoulder Stretch

• Sit tall with your feet level on the floor.
• Reach your right arm across your chest, holding it with your left hand.
• Hold for 15-30 seconds, feeling a stretch in your shoulder.
• Repeat on the opposite side.
• This exercise improves shoulder mobility and flexibility.

10. Seated Marching

• Sit on the edge of the chair, feet hip-width apart.
• Lift one leg toward your chest and then lower it.
• Repeat on the opposite leg, generating a marching motion.
• Continue for 1-2 minutes, focusing on controlled motions.
• Seated marching increases hip and knee mobility.
Perform these chair yoga movements on a regular basis, moving within a pain-free range of motion. Maintain smooth, controlled movements and

remember to breathe deeply throughout each exercise. Consult a healthcare expert before beginning a new fitness plan if you have any current health issues.

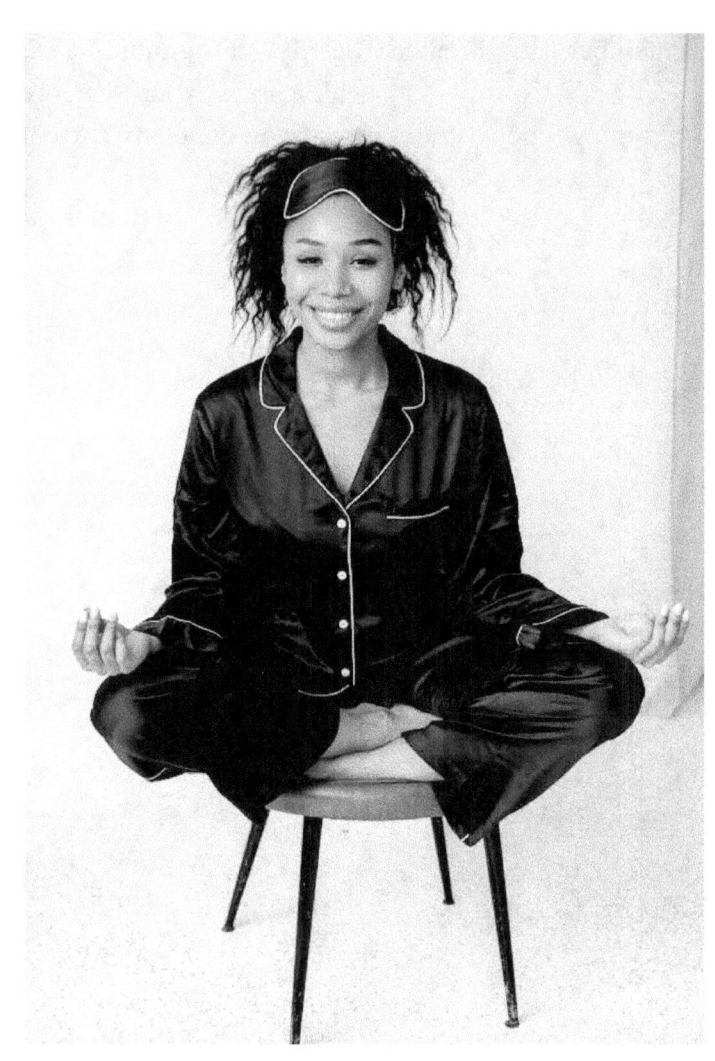

CHAPTER 6: BUILDING STRENGTH

1. Chair Squat with Leg Lift

• Sit on the edge of the chair, feet hip-width apart.
• Inhale and rise up, extending one leg to the side.
• Exhale and sink back into your chair.
• Repeat 10-12 times on each leg.
• This workout strengthens the legs and improves balance.

2. Seated Side Leg Lifts

• Sit tall with your back straight.
• Lift one leg to the side, engaging your outer hip.
• Hold for a few seconds, then lower it.
• Repeat 10-12 times on each leg.
• This workout focuses on the outside hips and thighs.

3. Chair Tricep Dips

• Sit on the chair's edge, hands on the seat.
• Slide your hips forward and lower your body.
• Bend your elbows to a 90-degree angle.
• Push back up with your palms.
• Repeat for 12-15 times.

• Tricep dips help to strengthen the arms and shoulders.

4. Seated Knee Extension

• Sit tall with your back straight.
• Extend one leg forward, using the quadriceps.
• Hold for a few seconds, then lower it.
• Repeat 10-12 times on each leg.
• This workout strengthens the quadriceps and enhances knee strength.

5. Seated Side Plank

• Sit on the chair's edge, right hand on the seat.
• Lift your hips, forming a straight line from head to heels.
• Hold for 15-30 seconds while activating your core.
• Lower your hips and move to the left side.
• Side planks strengthen the core and obliques.

6. Seated Bicep Curl

• Sit tall with your back straight.
• Hold a water bottle or small weights in each hand.
• Inhale and curl the weights towards your shoulders.
• Exhale and drop them back down.
• Repeat for 12-15 times.

• Bicep curls help to strengthen the arms.

7. Chair Warrior Pose

• Sit on the chair's edge, feet apart.
• Extend your right foot and bend your right knee.
• Extend your arms upward, palms facing each other.
• Hold for 15-30 seconds while working your leg muscles.
• Change sides.
• Chair Warrior Pose strengthens the legs and improves balance.

8. Seated Leg Press

• Sit up straight and comfortably.
• Wrap a resistance band across your legs.
• Push your legs outward against the resistance.
• Hold for a few seconds, then release.
• Repeat for 12-15 times.
• Leg presses work the inside thighs.

9. Seated Row

• Sit tall with a resistance band in front of you.
• Hold the ends of the band with both hands.
• Inhale and pull the band towards your chest.
• Exhale, then exhale again.

• Repeat for 12-15 times.
• Seated rows work the upper back and shoulders.

10. Seated Mountain Pose

• Sit with your feet flat on the floor.
• Inhale and lift your arms upwards, palms facing each other.
• Engage your core and hold for 15-30 seconds.
• Exhale and drop your arms.
• Seated Mountain Pose strengthens the arms, shoulders, and core.

Perform these chair yoga exercises on a daily basis, concentrating on perfect form and controlled movements. Consult a healthcare expert before beginning a new fitness regimen if you have any pre-existing health issues.

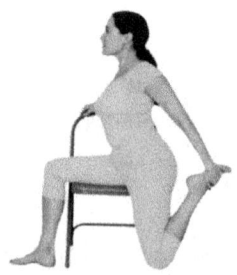

CHAPTER 7: BUILDING BALANCE

1. Seated Leg Cross

• Sit tall with your feet level on the floor.
• Cross your right foot over your left knee.
• Hold for 15-30 seconds while activating your core.
• Repeat on the opposite side.
• This exercise increases hip flexibility and balance.

2. Heel-to-Toe Rocks

• Sit on the chair's edge, with your feet flat on the floor.
• Lift your heels and balance on the balls of your feet.
• Rock forward onto your toes and backward onto your heels.
• Repeat for 12-15 rocks.
• This exercise improves ankle stability and balance.

3. Chair Tree Pose

• Sit with your back straight and your feet flat on the floor.

• Raise your right foot and place the sole against your inner left thigh.
• Hold for 15-30 seconds, finding a focal point for balance.
• Repeat on the opposite side.
• Chair Tree Pose strengthens the legs and improves balance.

4. Seated Eagle Arms

• Sit tall with your arms stretched in front of you.
• Cross your right arm across your left, entwining your forearms.
• Lift your elbows and lower your shoulders.
• Hold for 15-30 seconds, then swap arms.
• Seated Eagle Arms improve balance and attention.

5. Seated Warrior III

• Sit on the chair's edge, feet hip-width apart.
• Lean forward and straighten your right leg.
• Hold for 15-30 seconds, keeping your back straight.
• Rep on the opposite side.
• Seated Warrior III develops core strength and balance.

6. Seated Figure Four Stretch

• Sit with your feet flat on the floor.
• Cross your right ankle over your left knee.
• Hold for 15-30 seconds, feeling a stretch in the hip.
• Rep on the opposite side.
• This exercise improves hip flexibility and balance.

7. Seated Side Leg Extension

• Sit tall with your back straight.
• Extend one leg to the side.
• Hold for 15-30 seconds, activating your inner thigh.
• Repeat on the opposite side.
• This exercise strengthens the outer hips and improves balance.

8. Seated Warrior II

• Sit on the chair's edge, feet apart.
• Extend your right foot and bend your right knee.
• Extend your arms parallel to the floor.
• Hold for 15-30 seconds while working your leg muscles.
• Change sides.
• Seated Warrior II improves strength and balance.

9. Seated Side Plank with Leg Lift

• Sit on the chair's edge, supporting yourself with your right hand.
• Raise your hips, stretching your left leg to the side.
• Hold for 15-30 seconds while activating your core.
• Lower your hips and swap sides.
• This workout strengthens the core and improves balance.

10. Chair Toe Taps

• Sit tall with your feet flat on the floor.
• Lift your right foot and tap your toes on the floor.
• Repeat for 12-15 taps, then turn to the other foot.
• Chair toe taps increase ankle stability and balance.
Perform these chair yoga movements on a daily basis, paying close attention to perfect form and deep breathing. Consult a healthcare expert before beginning a new fitness regimen if you have any pre-existing health issues.

Safety Guidelines for Balance Exercises

Maintaining balance becomes increasingly crucial as we age. Chair yoga, with its reduced poses and firm support, is a gentle yet effective technique for seniors to improve balance and prevent falls. While the benefits are substantial, safety must always come first. When including balancing exercises into your chair yoga regimen, keep the following points in mind:

1. Select the Appropriate Chair:

A stable chair is an absolute must. Choose one with a robust base, armrests (optional), and a flat, firm seat. Avoid chairs with wheels or shaky legs.

2. Wear Supportive Shoes:

Get rid of your slippers! Wear comfortable shoes with non-slip soles to give traction and avoid slips.

3. Listen to Your Body:

Don't push yourself over your boundaries. Begin with basic postures and work your way up as you gain strength and confidence. If you feel any discomfort, dizziness, or unsteadiness, stop immediately and inform your doctor.

4. Warm-up and Cool-down:

Begin with mild motions to warm up your muscles and joints, like with any workout. Finish with some exercises to cool down and prevent injury.

5. Prioritize Quality Over Quantity:

It's not about how many times you can execute a posture; it's about executing it correctly. Maintain proper posture, engage your core, and keep your motions calm and controlled.

6. Modify as Needed:

Don't be scared to modify postures to suit your talents. If a posture feels too difficult, use props like cushions or blocks for added support, or simply sit and observe.

7. Relax:

Deep, regulated breathing improves balance and attention. Keep your breath in sync with your motions to be present and in touch with your body.

8. Be aware of your surroundings:

To prevent tripping dangers, practice in a clear, uncluttered area. Keep a neighboring wall handy for extra support if necessary.

9. Be Patient and Consistent:

Building balance requires time and practice. For the best results, be patient with yourself and continue to your chair yoga program on a daily basis.

10. Enjoy the Journey:

Concentrate on the enjoyment and sense of accomplishment, rather than the ultimate result. Celebrate your success, no matter how modest, and enjoy the journey of improving your balance and well-being via chair yoga.

CHAPTER 8: CARDIO EXERCISES

1. Seated Jumping Jacks

• Sit with your back straight and your feet flat on the floor.
• Inhale, raise your arms aloft, and lift your heels off the ground.
• Exhale, and simultaneously drop your arms and heels.
• Repeat for 30 seconds, increasing the intensity as needed.
• This workout raises the heart rate and supports cardiovascular health.

2. Seated Knee Taps

• Sit tall with your feet level on the floor.
• Lift one leg toward your chest and tap it with the opposing hand.
• Alternate between knees at a quick speed.
• Continue for 1-2 minutes, working the core and progressively increasing the tempo.
• Seated knee taps raise heart rate and leg strength.

3. Seated High Knees

• Sit with your back straight and your feet flat on the floor.
• Lift your right knee toward your chest, then switch to the left.
• Continue marching by alternating your legs.
• Perform for 1-2 minutes, gradually increasing pace.
• Seated high knees raise the heart rate and stimulate the abdominal muscles.

4. Chair Step-Ups

• Sit on the chair's edge, feet hip-width apart.
• Step one foot onto the chair, elevating your body slightly.
• Alternate between legs in a rapid, rhythmic motion.
• Continue for 1-2 minutes, simulating a step-up action.
• Chair step-ups offer an aerobic boost while also targeting the lower body.

5. Seated Running in Place

• Sit tall, with your feet floating over the floor.
• Lift and lower your legs in a running motion.

• Increase the tempo progressively while keeping a quick beat.
• Continue for 1-2 minutes, focusing on steady movement.
• Seated running improves cardiovascular endurance.

6. Seated Cross Body Punches

• Maintain a straight spine and engage your core.
• Punch your right arm across your body to the left side.
• Alternate between arms in a quick, controlled motion.
• Continue for 1-2 minutes, keeping the effort high.
• This workout raises the heart rate and works the upper body.

7. Seated Mountain Climbers

• Sit on the chair's edge, your hands holding the sides.
• Lift your knees toward your chest in a running motion.
• Increase the speed progressively, performing for 1-2 minutes.
• Seated mountain climbers give a full-body aerobic exercise.

8. Seated Fast Arm Circles

• Sit with your feet flat on the floor.
• Extend your arms to the sides.
• Rotate your arms in tiny, rapid circles.
• Continue for 1-2 minutes, increasing pace as tolerated.
• Fast arm circles increase heart rate and engage shoulder muscles.

9. Seated Tap Dance

• Sit with your feet flat on the floor.
• Tap your toes on the floor in a rhythmic fashion.
• Increase the pace gradually while keeping a steady rhythm.
• Perform for 1-2 minutes, focusing on the lower body and core.
• Seated tap dance is a fun and effective cardio workout.

10. Seated Cross Body Knee Strikes

• Sit tall and raise your right knee towards your left elbow.
• Alternate between knees in a rapid cross-body action.
• Continue at a quick speed for 1-2 minutes.
• Seated cross-body knee strikes raise heart rate and activate the core.

CHAPTER 9: CHAIR YOGA FOR WEIGHT LOSS

1. Seated Bicycle Crunches

• Sit with your back straight and your hands behind your head.
• Raise your right knee to your chest while bringing your left elbow to it.
• Switch sides in a smooth manner while activating your core.
• Perform 15-20 repetitions on each side.
• Seated bicycle crunches stimulate the abdominal muscles for a core workout.

2. Chair Squat with Twist

• Sit tall with your feet level on the floor.
• Inhale, stand up, and rotate your torso to the right.
• Exhale, return to the center, and sit back down.
• Twist to the left again.
• Perform 12-15 repetitions on each side.
• This workout focuses the core and works the obliques.

3. Seated Jump Rope

• Sit up straight and imagine yourself holding a jump rope.
• Lift your heels while rotating your wrists in a leaping motion.
• Increase the tempo progressively while keeping a quick pace.
• Continue for 1-2 minutes, simulating a jumping rope workout.
• Seated jump rope raises heart rate and assists in calorie burning.

4. Chair Leg Raises

• Sit on the edge of the chair, hands on the sides.
• Raise both legs straight in front of you.
• Lower them back down without contacting the floor.
• Perform 15-20 repetitions while activating the lower abdominal muscles.
• Chair leg lifts assist tone the lower abdomen and improve the core.

5. Seated Russian Twists

• Sit with your back straight and a water bottle or light weight in your hand.

• Lean back slightly, engage your core, and twist to one side.
• Return to the center and twist to the opposite side.
• Perform 15-20 twists on each side.
• Seated Russian twists tone the obliques and help with torso toning.

6. Seated Side Leg Lift and Reach

• Sit with your back straight and your legs out to the side.
• Lift one leg and stretch your opposing hand towards your toes.
• Lower the leg and swap sides.
• Perform 12-15 repetitions on each side.
• This exercise works the core, legs, and increases flexibility.

7. Chair Plank

• Sit on the chair's edge, lay your hands on the seat, and walk your feet back.
• Make a straight line from your head to your heels, engaging your core.
• Hold the plank posture for 30-60 seconds.
• The chair plank trains the entire body and helps to improve strength.

8. Seated Rowing

• Sit tall with a resistance band or modest weights.
• Extend your arms forward and draw the elbows back, compressing the shoulder blades.
• Repeat for 15-20 times.
• Seated rowing works the upper back, shoulders, and arms.

9. Seated High Kicks

• Sit with your back straight and your feet floating over the floor.
• Kick one leg up towards the ceiling while engaging your core.
• Alternate between legs in a quick, controlled motion.
• Perform for 1-2 minutes.
• Seated high kicks increase heart rate and engage the abdominal muscles.

10. Seated Mountain Climbers with Rotation

• Sit on the chair's edge with your hands on the seat.
• In a running action, lift your legs to your chest.
• Rotate your body, bringing one knee to the opposite elbow.
• Hold for 1-2 minutes, activating the core.
• This exercise mixes aerobic and core strengthening.

CHAPTER 10: MUSCLE TONING EXERCISES

1. Seated Shoulder Press

• Sit tall with a straight spine, holding light weights or water bottles in each hand.
• Inhale and lift your arms overhead.
• Exhale and drop them back down.
• Perform 15-20 repetitions.
• Seated shoulder presses work the deltoids and upper arms.

2. Seated Tricep Extension

• Sit with a straight back and one weight or water bottle in each hand.
• Exhale and raise your arms overhead.
• Exhale and bend your elbows, reducing the weight behind your head.
• Perform 15-20 repetitions.
• Seated tricep extensions train the triceps and enhance arm tone.

3. Seated Leg Curl

• Sit on the chair with your feet flat on the floor.
• Inhale and elevate one foot towards your glutes.

• Exhale and lower it back down.
• Repeat 15-20 times on each leg.
• Seated leg curls work the hamstrings and enhance leg muscular tone.

4. Chair Side Plank with Leg Lift

• Sit on the chair's edge, supporting yourself with your right hand.
• Raise your hips, stretching your left leg to the side.
• Hold for 15-30 seconds, activating your core and outer thighs.
• Lower your hips and swap sides.
• This workout works the core, obliques, and outer thighs.

5. Seated Bicep Twist

• Sit tall with a straight spine and a light weight or water bottle in each hand.
• Inhale and curl the weights towards your shoulders.
• Exhale and rotate your body to the right, working the obliques.
• Inhale back to the center and repeat on the left side.
• Perform 15-20 repetitions on each side.
• Seated bicep twists target the biceps and obliques.

6. Chair Calf Raises

• Sit with your feet flat on the floor.
• Inhale and raise your heels off the ground.
• Exhale and drop them back down.
• Perform 20-25 repetitions.
• Chair calf raises tone the calf muscles.

7. Seated Chest Opener

• Sit tall with your hands clasped behind your back.
• Inhale, elevate your chest, and press your shoulder blades together.
• Exhale and release.
• Perform 15-20 repetitions.
• Seated chest openers tone the chest and enhance posture.

8. Seated Lateral Raises

• Sit tall, holding light weights or water bottles in each hand.
• Inhale and lift your arms to your sides at shoulder height.
• Exhale and drop them back down.
• Perform 15-20 repetitions.
• Seated lateral raises work the deltoids and shoulder muscles.

9. Seated Hip Flexor Stretch with Knee Lift

• Maintain a straight spine while sitting.
• Inhale and bring your right knee to your chest.
• Exhale and lower it back down.
• Repeat 15-20 times on each leg.
• This workout strengthens and tones the hip flexors.

10. Chair Plank with Knee Tuck

• Sit on the edge of the chair, lay your hands on the seat, and walk your feet back.
• Make a straight line from head to heels.
• Inhale, tuck your right knee into your chest.
• Exhale and stretch the leg back.
• Switch to the left knee.
• Do 15-20 knee tucks on each leg.
• This workout tones the core, arms, and enhances general strength.

CHAPTER 11: RELAXATION & COOL DOWN EXERCISES

1. Seated Forward Bend with Gentle Neck Stretch

• Sit comfortably with your feet flat on the floor.
• Inhale and stretch your spine.
• Exhale, bend at the hips, and extend forward with your hands.
• Allow your head to hang softly, experiencing a stretch in your spine and neck.
• Hold for 30 seconds, inhaling deeply and relaxing into the stretch.

2. Chair Cat-Cow Stretch

• Sit with your spine straight and your hands on your knees.
• Inhale, arch your back, and elevate your chest (Cow pose).
• Exhale, circle your spine, and bring your chin to your chest (Cat pose).
• Repeat this pattern for 1-2 minutes, developing flexibility and relaxation.

3. Seated Side Stretch and Breath Awareness

• Sit with your feet flat on the floor.
• Inhale, lift your right arm above, and softly lean to the left.
• Exhale, experiencing a stretch down your right side.
• Hold for 30 seconds, focusing on deep, rhythmic breathing.
• Repeat on the opposite side.

4. Chair Twist with Gentle Neck Release

• Sit with your feet flat on the floor and your back straight.
• Inhale and rotate your body to the right, resting your left hand on your right knee.
• Exhale and move your head to the right for a slight neck stretch.
• Hold for 30 seconds before switching to the other side.

5. Seated Ankle Rolls with Mindful Breathing

• Sit comfortably with your hands on your knees.

• Lift one foot off the floor and spin your ankle in a circular manner.
• Breathe deeply and mindfully as you move.
• Perform for 1-2 minutes, then switch to the other ankle.

6. Chair Butterfly Stretch

• Sit with your back straight and your feet together.
• Inhale and stretch your spine.
• Exhale and softly press your knees to the floor, experiencing a stretch in your inner thighs.
• Hold for 30 seconds, concentrating on calm breathing.

7. Seated Heart Opener

• Sit tall with your hands clasped behind your back.
• Inhale, elevate your chest, and press your shoulder blades together.
• Exhale, allowing your shoulders to relax.
• Hold for 30 seconds, opening up the chest and encouraging relaxation.

8. Chair Child's Pose

• Sit in the chair with your knees open and your toes touching.

• Inhale and stretch your arms forward, lowering your chest to the floor.
• Exhale while resting your forehead on the chair seat.
• Hold for 30 seconds, relieving tension in the lower back and shoulders.

9. Seated Neck and Shoulder Rolls

• Sit comfortably with your feet flat on the floor.
• Inhale and elevate your shoulders towards your ears.
• Exhale and roll your shoulders back and down.
• Perform moderate neck rolls in both directions.
• Repeat for 1-2 minutes, reducing tension in the neck and shoulders.

10. Chair Meditation

• Sit with your back straight and your hands on your knees.
• Close your eyes and concentrate on your breath.
• Inhale deeply while counting to four, then exhale gently.
• Continue for 5-10 minutes, allowing your thoughts to calm and fostering total relaxation.

CHAPTER 12: MINDFUL EATING PRACTICES FOR SENIORS

Consider a balanced diet with portion management for weight loss. Put an emphasis on natural meals, lean meats, vegetables, and healthy fats. An anti-inflammatory diet rich in fruits, vegetables, whole grains, nuts, and fatty fish can help with flexibility and inflammation. Before making large dietary changes, contact a healthcare practitioner. Here's a list of diets that may aid in weight loss, flexibility, and inflammation reduction, along with a brief description of each and how to prepare it:

1. Quinoa and Vegetable Stir-Fry

Ingredients:
Quinoa, mixed veggies (bell peppers, broccoli, carrots), tofu or chicken.
Mode of Preparation:
• Cook quinoa according per package directions.
• Sauté veggies and protein of choice in olive oil.
• Season the quinoa and veggies with soy sauce.
Nutritional Values:
Calories: 400 kcal, Protein: 18g, Fiber: 8g.

2. Salmon and Avocado Salad

Ingredients:
Grilled salmon, mixed greens, cherry tomatoes, and avocado.

Mode of Preparation:
• Grill the salmon and allow it to cool.
• Toss greens, cherry tomatoes, and avocado together.
• Top with flaked salmon.

Nutritional Values:
Calories: 350 kcal, Protein: 25g, Omega-3: 1.5g.

3. Sweet Potato and Chickpea Buddha Bowl

Ingredients:
Roasted sweet potatoes, chickpeas, quinoa, and spinach.

Mode of Preparation:
• Roast the sweet potatoes and chickpeas.
• Assemble with cooked quinoa and fresh spinach.

Nutritional Values:
Calories: 380 kcal, Protein: 15g, Fiber: 12g.

4. Mango and Shrimp Summer Rolls

Ingredients:
Rice paper, shrimp, mango, cucumber, and mint leaves.

Mode of Preparation:
• Soak rice paper in warm water.
• Fill with shrimp, mango, cucumber, and mint leaves.

Nutritional Values:
Calories: 250 kcal, Protein: 18g, Vitamin C: 30mg.

5. Mushroom and Spinach Omelette

Ingredients:
Eggs, mushrooms, spinach, and feta cheese.

Mode of Preparation:
• Sauté the mushrooms and spinach.
• Whisk the eggs and pour over the vegetables in a pan.
• Top with feta cheese.

Nutritional Values:
Calories: 280 kcal, Protein: 20g, Calcium: 150mg.

6. Lentil and Vegetable Soup

Ingredients:
Lentils, carrots, celery, onions, vegetable broth.
Mode of Preparation:
• Sauté veggies, then add lentils and broth.
• Simmer until the lentils are soft.
Nutritional Values:
Calories: 200 kcal, Protein: 12g, Fiber: 8g.

7. Turkey and Quinoa Stuffed Bell Peppers

Ingredients:
Ground turkey, quinoa, bell peppers, and tomatoes.
Mode of Preparation:
• Cook the quinoa and brown the turkey first.
• Fill bell peppers with the mixture and bake.
Nutritional Values:
Calories: 320 kcal, Protein: 22g, Fiber: 6g.

8. Greek Yogurt Parfait

Ingredients:
Greek yogurt, berries, oats, honey.
Mode of Preparation:
• Layer Greek yogurt, berries, and granola.
• Drizzle with honey.

Nutritional Values:
Calories: 250 kcal, Protein: 15g, Fat: 0g

9. Cauliflower Rice and Vegetable Bowl

Ingredients:
Cauliflower rice, mixed veggies (zucchini, bell peppers), grilled chicken.
Mode of Preparation:
• Sauté cauliflower rice and veggies.
• Top with grilled chicken.
Nutritional Values:
Calories: 280 kcal, Protein: 20g, Fiber: 10g.

10. Pesto Zoodles with Cherry Tomatoes

Ingredients:
Zucchini noodles, cherry tomatoes, pesto sauce.
Mode of Preparation:
• Spiralize zucchini to make noodles.
• Sauté zoodles with cherry tomatoes and pesto.
Nutritional Values:
Calories: 230 kcal, Protein: 8g, Healthy Fats: 15g.

11. Chia Seed Pudding with Berries:

Ingredients:
Chia seeds, almond milk, and mixed berries.
Mode of Preparation:
• Combine chia seeds and almond milk in a bowl and refrigerate overnight.
• Before serving, top with mixed berries.
Nutritional Values:
Calories: 180 kcal, protein: 5g, omega-3: 3g.

12. Caprese Salad Skewers

Ingredients:
Cherry tomatoes, mozzarella balls, fresh basil, and balsamic glaze.
Mode of Preparation:
• Thread tomatoes, mozzarella, and basil onto skewers.
• Drizzle with balsamic glaze.
Nutritional Values:
Calories: 220 kcal, Protein: 12g, Calcium: 300mg.

13. Eggplant and Tomato Stacks

Ingredients:
Eggplant slices, tomatoes, fresh mozzarella, basil.

Mode of Preparation:
• Grill eggplant slices and top with tomatoes and mozzarella.
• Garnish with fresh basil if desired.
Nutritional Values:
 Calcium: 260 kcal, Protein: 10g, and Fiber: 9g.

14. Markdown on Smoked Salmon and Cream

Ingredients:
Smoked salmon, whole grain wrap, cream cheese, cucumber slices.
Mode of Preparation:
• Spread cream cheese on the wrap, then stack with smoked salmon and cucumber.
• Roll and slice.
Nutritional Values:
Calories: 280 kcal, protein: 28g, Omega-3: 2.5g.

15. Sandwich with Almond Butter and Banana on Sale

Ingredients:
Whole grain bread, almond butter, banana slices.
Mode of Preparation:
• Spread almond butter over bread
• Add banana slices, and construct a sandwich.

Nutritional Values:
Calories: 320 kcal, Protein: 8g, Fiber: 6g.
These meals provide a choice of nutrient-dense options for seniors practicing chair yoga, supporting mindful eating and general well-being. Adjust portion sizes according to individual nutritional needs, and get individualized guidance from a healthcare practitioner.

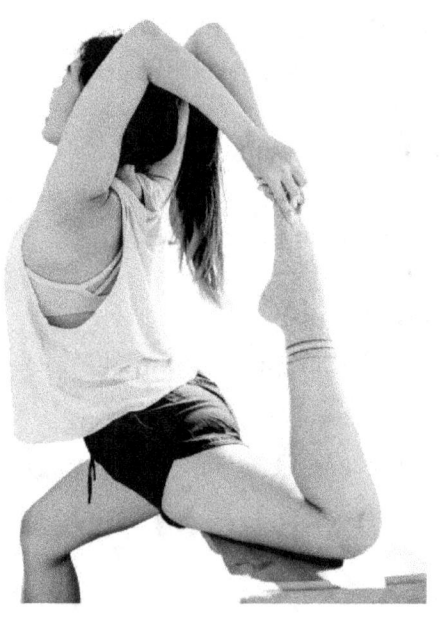

CONCLUSION

As you finish "Chair Yoga for Seniors Over 60," a pleasant sense of success floods over you. You've begun a voyage of self-discovery, 10 minutes at a time. This book was more than simply a compilation of exercises; it was a spark, promising restored balance, improved mobility, and even a lighter frame.

Remember how nervous you were at first? Perhaps your joints creaked in protest, your muscles unaccustomed to the need to move. But you felt a change with each guided stance and focused breath. The tightness dissipated, the muscles reacted, and within a spark of renewed strength erupted.

You recovered space in your body with each gentle stretch, reconnecting with muscles you'd forgotten about. You created rainbows with your arms, danced with your toes, and uncovered a secret resilience that was just waiting to emerge. Your ten-minute commitment became into a daily self-care routine, a quiet discussion with your body communicated via movement.

The book was about more than simply the physical. It was a portal to happiness and life. You regained your lively personality as you learnt to skillfully negotiate the positions. Laughter blended with deep breaths, grins formed on your lips, and a sense of lightheartedness returned.

"Chair Yoga for Seniors Over 60" wasn't a magical elixir, but it did have the components for a profound change. It demonstrated that age is simply a number and that movement, in all of its manifestations, is the language of regeneration. You chipped away at restrictions with each posture, replacing them with alternatives.

Don't let the adventure finish as you close the book. Allow the echoes of the positions to reverberate inside you as you go about your day. Step into the chair, take a deep breath, and appreciate the gift of mobility. You've discovered a powerful new weapon: your own body, which is eager to dance, bend, and prosper.

Remember, it only takes 10 minutes to rekindle the spark of happiness. You are the story's author, and "Chair Yoga for Seniors Over 60" has given you the pen. Continue writing, flowing, and finding delight in every soft movement. Your colorful dance, step by mindful stride, pose by mindful posture, awaits the world.

And on days when uncertainty creeps in, tell yourself, "I am over 60, yes, but I am also boundless."

Go forth and enjoy your life, dear reader!

WORKOUT PLANNER

My workout planner

DATE

DAY	ACTIVITIES	TIME	REMARK
DAY:1			
DAY:2			
DAY:3			
DAY:4			
DAY:5			
DAY:6			

NOTES

My workout planner

DAY	ACTIVITIES	TIME	REMARK
DAY:1			
DAY:2			
DAY:3			
DAY:4			
DAY:5			
DAY:6			

NOTES

My workout planner

DATE

DAY	ACTIVITIES	TIME	REMARK
DAY:1			
DAY:2			
DAY:3			
DAY:4			
DAY:5			
DAY:6			

NOTES

My workout planner

DAY	ACTIVITIES	TIME	REMARK
DAY:1			
DAY:2			
DAY:3			
DAY:4			
DAY:5			
DAY:6			

NOTES

www.ingramcontent.com/pod-product-compliance
Lightning Source LLC
Chambersburg PA
CBHW071103290526
45795CB00004B/1627